Skill in Action

Radicalizing Your Yoga Practice to Create a Just World

Michelle Cassandra Johnson

Copyright 2017 Michelle Cassandra Johnson
Published by Radical Transformation Media
Portland, Oregon
Cover concept and design by Ivan Moy
Cover Art by Ivan Moy
About the Author Photo Credit: Courtney Long
Printed in the United States of America

This book is dedicated to my grandmother's grandmothers. This book is dedicated to all of the social justice workers who are trying to make this world a better place. Skill in Action is dedicated to everyone who embodies an open-heart and a warrior spirit.

We are the ones we've been waiting for.

ACKNOWLEDGMENTS

First, I want to acknowledge Jeffrey Herrick. He has been my biggest cheerleader. He has supported me in so many ways and this book is no exception. He said, "yes" when I asked him to go to Kenya with me for the first time to volunteer with the Africa Yoga Project. That project birthed my decision to lead a teacher training on social justice and yoga. The inception of the teacher training led one of my trainees to suggest that I write a book about the process of merging social justice and yoga. This book is the result of that suggestion. I acknowledge the support I have received from my yoga teacher trainees. Three years ago, they entrusted me with their hearts, allowing me to lead them through a process of understanding the intersection of social justice and yoga.

Much of what I write in this book comes from my experiences as a yoga teacher, social worker and Dismantling Racism trainer. I thank my yoga community and all of the students who have shown up again and again because they feel called to something bigger than themselves. I thank my clients who commit to a process of self-exploration and trust me with their deepest, darkest secrets. In so many ways they have shown me how to bring things into the light. I acknowledge all of my colleagues with Dismantling Racism Works. You have trained me up, radicalized me and pushed me to use my voice even when I am afraid. Thank you Tema Okun, Cristina Rivera Chapman, Jonathan Henderson, Jes Kelley, Cynthia Brown, Kenneth Jones and Vivette Jeffries Logan. Much of what is written in this book comes from my experience of holding space for other beings. Thank you for teaching me how to hold space in a way that allowed me to recognize your truth and my own. Thank you for participating in the workshops, the classes and diving deep into "heart" work.

Thank you to my goddess circle, you have held me through transitions and assisted me in manifesting my dreams. Amy Burtaine is my best friend. She moved across the country a year ago and somehow she transmuted all time and space to continue to show up as my best friend. We are sisters for life and she believes in me, always and forever. Last but not least, thank you to my mother, Clara Johnson. It is only through her tenacity and life force that I am able to be fully alive today. She doesn't always understand my decisions but she does understand my heart. She tells me that she is proud of me all of the time and she taught me that I am limitless. Even though I am confined to this human experience in my black, female identified body, Clara always told me to dream big and make my dreams become reality.

TABLE OF CONTENTS

PREFACE

Where I'm From

I'm from Clara and Cornelius, a warrior mama and a contradiction for a papa.

I'm from the afterbirth, which came out before me and the baby boy my mama miscarried two years before having me.

I'm from the nurse pulling me out because I was losing oxygen and immobile, unwilling to enter this brutal and beautiful world.

I'm from 2 pounds and 3 ounces of strength and a full head of hair, fingernails and underdeveloped lungs.

I'm from asthma, Primatene mist and nebulizer treatments.

I'm from being away from my mother and father for the first nine days of my life.

I'm from hospital lights, loud sounds and various nurses picking me up and checking my vitals.

I'm from Dorothy and Fred, summers spent in their yard playing the stoplight game, making vanilla milkshakes, mud pies and picking hydrangeas from my grandmother's backyard.

I'm from Whitewood Road, the man in the mirror, my guardian angel and the yellow wallpaper in a kitchen that was always full of laughter, noise- life.

I'm from Madonna, Michael, Duran Duran, MC Hammer, Purple Rain and Joan Armatrading.

I'm from being the only black girl in my class and "you're not like the other kids, Michelle."

I'm from private school, "you talk white, you dress white", and "do you think you're white?"

I'm from do the best that you can, you are black and beautiful and "show them who you really are, Michelle."
I'm from the loneliness, not fitting in, confusion of what it meant to live in the middle of black and white.
I'm from being awake, at a very young age, seeing the ways of the world that made no sense to me but that let me know suffering is real, it happens across color lines and it is killing people.
I'm from wanting to create a world where everyone can move in physical space, freely, without fear.
I'm from liberation, yours and mine, ours.
I'm from the breath, each inhale and exhale.
I am from you and you are from me.

I came to yoga by way of the breath.

When someone has experienced trauma, the breath is the most useful resource to stabilize the nervous system. The breath sends a signal that all is well; everything is okay. In a culture that would rather my black body not exist, let alone breathe, this feeling of "all is well" has been more than illusive. From the moment that I took my first breath until now, I have been on a journey to find air, to create an expansive inhale and a deepening of experience with my exhale. This is how I found it:

My birth story begins with a watermelon. After a craving got the best of her, my mother put a rusty Radio Flyer wagon in the trunk of her car and drove to the grocery store. After finding the perfect one, rolling it onto the wagon and then into her car, she felt accomplished. But before she could taste the sweet fruit of her labor, her water broke. After two long days of laboring, a nurse pressed on her belly and said, "Your baby is small." The doctor added, "The baby is losing oxygen, we have to act fast." She was placed on a cold table and asked to count down from 10 to one, only to wake up having delivered a baby by C-section who was nowhere to be found.

For the first nine days of my life, I lived in an incubator, hooked up to tubes and monitored by doctors and nurses when I should have been connecting with my mama. My father was primarily absent and only came when called by Child Protection Services.

As a black woman in the 1970s, partnered with what was perceived as an absentee father, my mother was a parent to one adopted, biracial boy and now a new parent to a premature child who had a unibrow, a full head of hair and fingernails, and underdeveloped lungs.

At the age of four, I was diagnosed with asthma, following in the footsteps of both of my parents. When I watched my father use his Primatene mist, sucking in medicine to make his lungs properly work, I wondered why he needed something to help him breathe. My mother listened for my breath and when she could hear my wheezing from three rooms over, she would rush in and say, "Do you need to go to the hospital?" I would always resist, thinking that I could power through the elephant seated proudly on my chest. Soon I understood that the elephant was determined to collapse my lungs, so I would tell my mom that it was time to go to the hospital.

It wasn't until college that I was prescribed an inhaler that allowed me access to fuller, deeper breaths. Many years later, I am still using it. But college wasn't all deep breathing. I had become keenly aware of oppression, racism and white supremacy. I was a black girl at a mostly white college in Colonial Williamsburg. I didn't fit into the Black Student Movement because I wasn't "black enough" and I didn't fit in with the white students because I am not white. So, I stood somewhere between, trying to find my footing and the grey zone.

I was first introduced to yoga in college. I remember being the only black girl in our fitness class practicing yoga. My understanding of oppression and privilege made me feel disembodied. That yoga class was not a space for affirmation, validation or spiritual transformation. I left that fitness class and college lacking a deeper connection with my body, mind, heart and spirit. I graduated college in three years to allay the burden of my mother having to pay off an even larger student loan.

During my first semester in graduate school at the University of North Carolina's School of Social Work, my breath was taken away in an entirely different context: I was sexually assaulted. I'm not sure how I graduated, I'm not sure how I passed any of my classes but in 1998 grace shone down on me and allowed me to graduate with my Masters of Social Work. I remember learning in textbooks about experiences that I had first hand, particularly in the Confronting Oppression class. After graduating, and learning about the reality of many people's lives from textbooks, I set out to be a school social worker in Chapel Hill, NC.

In 2009, I met Lori Burgwyn, Franklin Street Yoga Studio owner, who introduced me to the ujjayi breath, a victorious breath. I felt alive in a way that I hadn't since before I was sexually assaulted in graduate school. I felt every cell, muscle, bone, heartbeat and breath. Using this breath, I began the ongoing work of becoming and remaining both a yoga teacher and a student.

Before becoming a yoga teacher, I was a social worker. I spent many sessions with individual clients and groups talking about the mind body connection. At one point, I remember being in session describing breathing techniques and realizing that I could just show my client how to breathe fully so that she could experience more space and liberation in her body and psyche. From that point on, I knew that I wanted to merge body awareness and healing with psychotherapy and social justice work. My experience as a black woman living in a culture that is wedded to white supremacy led me to become a social worker. My experience of being forced to disconnect from my body to survive led me to become a social justice activist. My longing for liberation in my body and beyond led me to become a yogi. My understanding of how social change occurs led me to merge social justice and yoga.

One must be connected with their breath to feel their body. A connection to the body allows one to feel their heart. A connection with the heart allows one to become clear about their values so that they may connect with their humanity. When one sees their own humanity and realizes that others are suffering around them they have the opportunity to connect with the oneness of all beings and our shared humanity. From the breath, body, heart and awareness of humanity, one must take action. No one can exist without taking action. Skill in Action.

Introduction

S kill in Action has its roots in the ancient text of the Bhaga-vad Gita. In 2011, my dear friend and social justice com-rade Claudia Horwitz introduced me to this powerful sto-ry as we co-taught a workshop titled, "Yoga for Social Change." The Bhagavad Gita is a classical yogic text in which a warrior, Arjuna, is guided by Krishna and is prodded and pushed to live into his dharma, or duty, which happened to be fighting a war. Arjuna is asked to fight his friends and family and this call to duty makes no sense to him. He tries to find ways out of the conflict and Krishna keeps on pushing him back into the war, his higher purpose, and his duty. Krishna is teaching Ar-juna about his ego, evil, conflict, war, difference, discipline and grace. Arjuna finally surrenders to his dharma. Krishna invites Arjuna to lean into the understanding that God lives within him, the Divine spark and spirit is in all of us and we are the oneness of being.

I distinctly remember when I heard "we are all one." I was a little irritated at the notion that we are seen as one when my re-ality as a black woman in the world was so counter to being seen at all. A premature black baby with underdeveloped lungs and an impending diagnosis of asthma, separated from her mother, with what was perceived as an absentee father. I knew that my lived experience didn't reflect the oneness of all beings.

Claudia followed up the idea that we are one by sharing two verses from the Gita-

"On this path no effort is wasted, no gain ever reversed, for even a little bit of this practice will shelter you from sorrow."

And, "Yoga is Skill in Action. Do every action to the best of your ability."

I remember getting chills when I heard the words "yoga is skill in action." It sounds simple, but it is a conversation that is absent in many discussions or practices of yoga in the Western Hemisphere. Most yoga spaces do not teach that yoga is an action and a skill to be used to guide us in the world. The Gita offers the perfect pairing of our call to action: the urgency around living into our dharma and how to use the practice of yoga as a guide to meet the call to action for the collective good.

Skill in Action: Radicalizing Your Yoga Practice to Create a Just World will ask you to explore the deeply transformational practice of yoga, and to become a social change agent so that you can create a world that is just for all. This book explores liberation for ourselves and others, while asking us to engage in our own agency, whether that manifests as activism, volunteer work, or changing our relationships with others and ourselves.

Skill in Action clearly defines power and privilege, oppression, liberation and suffering, and will invite you to take steps to make changes in your life to create a world that allows all of us to be free. The end of each chapter includes a sample practice so that you can put this wisdom into action in your daily life. These sample practices include: breathwork, asana, meditation and interpersonal relational work.

In an effort to move toward liberation for all, the practices extend beyond the individual to offer resources and tools to shift institutional policies and procedures in a culture that has left all of us negatively impacted by white supremacy.

It is my hope that Skill in Action calls you and your community to take action and to not become complicit via complacency. It asks that we take the powerful practice of yoga and use it to create a world that makes space for all, that values all and that speaks truth to power.

Shared Language

Language is a powerful tool. Working for justice requires a clear understanding of various terms. For example, in my work leading Dismantling Racism trainings, we spend a great deal of time defining terms so that the participants have shared language to create their race equity goals. As you utilize this workbook, I want you to have a clear understanding of words and terms so that you can create clear goals focused on creating a just world. Most of the definitions offered here, are informed by critical race theory and scholars who have been studying and exploring racism and oppression for the whole of their lives.

Oppression

Oppression is the subjugation of one group of people to elevate another group of people. Often it involves violence but isn't limited to physical violence. It can include emotional, mental, spiritual and psychic violence as well.

Privilege

Privilege is the societal benefits bestowed upon people socially, politically and economically. Privilege can be based on race, class, age, ability level, mental health status, gender identity and sex.

White supremacy

White supremacy is an ideology and belief system that is based on a hierarchy of constructed racial categorizations where white is at the top, black is at the bottom and everyone else is between white and black. Dominant culture conditions us to believe that white supremacy should only be applied to hateful individuals or hate groups such as the Ku Klux Klan. It is important to understand that white supremacy is a belief system that perpetuates the idea that white is superior.

Racism

Racism is racial prejudice + social and institutional power
Racism is advantage based on race
Racism is oppression based on race
Racism is a white supremacy system

Suffering

In many religious or faith traditions, including Buddhism and Hinduism, understanding the afflictions that cause suffering inspires a deeper exploration of how we create a space of ultimate liberation and freedom. Given the historical legacy of war, violence, oppression, socially and politically constructed categories to minimize people and make them be seen as subhuman, and the privileging of groups of people at the expense of others, it is important to broaden the definition of suffering to move beyond the individual. Social and political forces have caused collective pain and cultural trauma and have normalized things that are absolutely absurd like the amount of children that go to bed hungry at night or the amount of black and brown bodies that are murdered at the hands of police whom are supported by a criminal justice system that chooses to serve and protect some and to annihilate others. Suffering is the experience of pain and distress psychically, emotionally, physically, mentally and spiritually.

Liberation

As with the definition of suffering, many religious and faith traditions including Buddhism and Hinduism focus on the pathway to enlightenment coming through freeing ourselves of our attachments to afflictions (our own suffering) and shifting our consciousness such that we can be free regardless of the circumstances.

In Man's Search for Meaning, Victor Frankel discusses the space between what was happening to him and what was within his power to change these conditions. He describes the physical and psychological experience of being in a concentration camp and his response was, "Between stimulus and response there is a space. In that space is our power to choose our response. In our response lies our growth and our freedom." Victor Frankel is correct, from a psychic perspective our freedom does live between what is happening to us, the stimulus and our response. Liberation is understanding our humanity and being able to see the humanity in others such that we understand our freedom is dependent upon others freedom.

Approach and Assumptions

It's important to be clear about my perspective and to communicate it with others as I engage in anti-racism and social justice work. These assumptions derive from a collaboration with my colleagues at Dismantling Racism Works, dRWorks. Many social justice warriors have put their energy into creating these assumptions:

- We live in a toxic culture that affects us all. We are not encouraged to see it, so we must learn to see our culture and how it teaches us to make transform the absurd into normal.

- Intention is not the same as impact. We just need to understand that we can have good intentions and still have a hurtful or damaging impact.

- Analyzing and cultivating awareness is a lifelong process. We all have questions, I hope to address some of your questions throughout the book, and my hope/assumption is that once you complete this book you will have more questions at a deeper level.

- I'm offering this book as a way of understanding how social justice intersects with yoga to radicalize the practice of yoga, individually and collectively. I understand that by sharing an analysis focused on social justice, racism and yoga, I risk reproducing racism by asking people already deeply traumatized to revisit and reflect on that trauma.

- We operate in a culture that assumes social justice, race equity and civil rights are for the benefit of the people being most oppressed in our culture. It is important to understand that injustice, racism, and a lack of civil rights affects us all and the work of understanding how is important for everyone.

- We have to develop awareness of ourselves and of our communities and of the world both as individuals and in community; we have to work together to love ourselves into who we are.

- We have to believe in the possibilities of creating the world we want to see by walking our talk and learning from our mistakes.

- None of this is easy and we have to do it anyway.

Radicalizing Your Yoga Practice to Create a Just World

Every social justice warrior that I know must be prepared for the journey. This particular journey requires three objects:

1. Please get a private journal that you will use to record reflections as you explore the intersection of social justice and your yogic path. This journal will serve as a space for you to record thoughts, feelings, awakenings and ideas.

2. Please create a space in your home, car, office, or within a natural landscape (a park, favorite mountain or ocean) to practice the meditations and breath practices offered throughout the book. It's simple. You don't need a yoga mat, or props, you just need a space where you can breathe, sit, tune into your inner wisdom and allow.

3. Lastly, I would encourage you to find an object that represents what creating a just world means to you. Choose an object that is meaningful to you. An object that represents freedom for all beings everywhere. You will place this object in a location where you will see it daily to remind you of your call to action and commitment to radicalizing your practice.

Poem for South African Women

Our own shadows disappear as the feet of thousands
by the tens of thousands pound the fallow land
into new dust that
rising like a marvelous pollen will be fertile
even as the first woman whispering
imagination to the trees around her made
for righteous fruit
from such deliberate defense of life
as no other still
will claim inferior to any other safety
in the world

The whispers too they
intimate to the inmost ear of every spirit
now aroused they
carousing in ferocious affirmation
of all peaceable and loving amplitude
sound a certainly unbounded heat
from a baptismal smoke where yes
there will be fire

And the babies cease alarm as mothers
raising arms
and heart high as the stars so far unseen
nevertheless hurl into the universe
a moving force
irreversible as light years
traveling to the open
eye

And who will join this standing up
and the ones who stood without sweet company
will sing and sing
back into the mountains and   .
if necessary
even under the sea

we are the ones we have been waiting for

-June Jordan

CHAPTER 1

WHAT IS SKILL IN ACTION?

Skill in Action is a way of life that illustrates what it means to live yoga for the transformation and liberation of all beings. It is an analysis of yoga that accounts for institutional and cultural forms of oppression while holding liberation at the heart of the practice. It is about feeling the connection between all beings and taking steps to serve the collective good with a goal of justice for all. It asks yoga practitioners and social change agents to take the benefits and lessons that come from a contemplative practice and to use their power to influence the world.

The Cultural Context

It is 2017 and we are living in a world that encompasses "Trump's America" on the heels of eight years of the first and likely ever black family in the white house. Right after Obama was elected for his first term as President of the United States, my father would get the biggest kick out of saying, "I never thought there would be afro sheen in the White House." What my father was really saying was that "White" America was going to lose their mind because black people inhabited spaces that were created and destined for white people. I have lost count of the amount of black and brown people who have been murdered at the hands of police, white vigilantes and people who will protect their right to bear arms because they live in a culture of fear that will protect their white power to no end.

In 2016, I had many conversations with white people who didn't believe that Trump could become president. The people I spoke to put far too much stock into humanity.

I was out to dinner with a friend on the night of the election. We watched the returns and I remember eating a bite of my fried chicken and arugula and thinking, this isn't looking good. I came home, went to sleep and woke up at 1:00 a.m. only to see that the nightmare I was having was actually reality. I texted a friend to say, "What is going on, what happened?" He replied and said, "white people." I texted back and said, "Yes, white people."

"First they came for the Socialists and I did not speak out-

Because I am not a Socialist.

Then they came for the Trade Unionists, and I did not speak out-

Because I was not a Trade Unionist.

Then they came for the Jews, and I did not speak out-

Because I am not a Jew.

Then they came for me-and there was not one left to speak for me"

— *Martin Niemöller*

When the election results were confirmed, I cried, I prayed and I sat in my bed and thought, "We are going to perish." Then I remembered my 95-year-old grandmother, Dorothy, who has survived plenty of Donald Trumps and I began to trust that some of us would be able to survive.

"And when the sun rises we are afraid it might not remain

when the sun sets we are afraid it might not rise

in the morning when our stomachs are full we are afraid of indigestion

when our stomachs are empty we are afraid we may never eat again

when we are loved we are afraid love will vanish

when we are alone we are afraid love will never return

and when we speak we are afraid our words will not be heard nor welcomed

but when we are silent we are still afraid

So it is better to speak remembering we were never meant to survive."

— Audre Lorde, The Black Unicorn

Many of us women of color weren't ever meant to survive and that reality seems to be more apparent now that we have a President who has appointed white supremacists to his cabinet. Eric Garner, "I cannot breathe", Trayvon Martin a boy child going to the store to get candy, and Sandra Bland, a woman who could have been me wasn't enough to awaken us. Freddie Gray who died rolling around in the back of a police van, Tamir Rice another boy child playing with a toy gun murdered by police who have been conditioned to see him as a dangerous black man wasn't enough to awaken us. And so many others weren't enough for people to wake up to the reality of injustice in a country that is anything but post-racial. We are living in a country in a culture where islamophobia, transphobia, racism, sexism, sexual assault and police brutality have been normalized.

I remember the night when George Zimmerman was acquitted for killing Trayvon Martin, July 14, 2013. I had been out to dinner at the same restaurant where I sat during our 2016 Presidential election. I came home from dinner, read Facebook and fell to the floor. It was as if the ancestral trauma was moving in, up and out of me like bile -- dry heaving emotionally and energetically. That night marked a time for me when something cracked open, something cracked open, or rather shattered. Something shifted and since then, I haven't been the same. I cried all evening and I couldn't rest or sleep because the tectonic plates had shifted under my feet and in my consciousness. A whole new continent and reality were being formed.

Life and Death

Our natural state is that of feeling our breath flowing in and out, deeply and fully. And yet, we are in a time where people are struggling to literally and figuratively find a way to breathe. Dominant culture asks us to disconnect from our humanity, our bodies, and our wholeness while buying into a narrative stating that some of us are meant to be free while others are meant to suffer.

The experience of being a black person in a whitewashed America takes away my breath. The experience of seeing people who look just like me, black, female, young, and ambitious being murdered at the hands of police and white supremacy takes my breath away. Liberation and freedom, our natural state (according to the yogic path) are about our capacity to breathe freely, which translates into our capacity to move freely while navigating institutions and cultural landscapes that we did not define individually or collectively.

Not being able to define your reality takes the breath away. Being told that there is a level playing field when you don't even know that there is a field, starting line or way to gain an advantage, takes away the breath. Being conditioned to believe that you are inferior as a person, inhibiting your ability to have a fair chance at a job, housing, a bank loan, equitable education for your family and yourself takes away the breath. Being conditioned to believe that we are post-racial, that we have transcended the conditions that enslaved my great grandmother Angie, and liberated me because I was privileged enough to have access to an education that afforded me the right to try to fight injustice from within the system takes away the breath. Oppression takes the breath away. And when we aren't breathing, when we are unable to reach a state of reorganization and homeostasis, we die. Some yogis believe that we should think about our death everyday. That we should recognize with each passing moment that we are dying so that we might change the way that we live.

We are dying, we need to change the way that we are living.

A New Way of Living

Yoga means to "yolk." It means bringing together things that seem to be in opposition like our mind and body or our heart and spirit. Yoga gives us the opportunity to show up and practice again and again, to start over. We are living in a time where we need to begin again. The practice of yoga teaches us to act skillfully and radically, moving us beyond the borders of our individual minds, hearts, bodies and spirits.

The practice of yoga offers principles and guidelines that instruct us on how to take skillful and radical action. Many of these principles are based on the ancient yogic text, the Yoga Sutras. Sutra means to string or thread and the yoga sutras, comprised of four different chapters, includes 196 Indian Sutras.

I will focus on two tenants of the 8-limbed path of yoga, the Yamas and Niyamas. The yamas and niyamas will guide you on your life's journey and yogic path. The yamas focus on our interactions with others and the niyamas focus on our inner world and our relationship with self.

Yamas and Niyamas: Ethical Foundation of Yoga

Yamas: Ethical behavior towards others

Ahimsa: non violence, non harming through actions, thoughts, and words

Ahimsa is the absence of injustice, violence and cruelty. This includes actions, words and ways of living. Ahimsa means always behaving in a way that takes into account if behavior is causing harm or injustice.

Satya: truthfulness

Satya means, "to speak the truth." Dominant culture perpetuates the belief that there is one narrative. Moving beyond the idea that only one truth exists allows us to create space for dialogue, authenticity, learning, opening and understanding.

Asteya: non-stealing, not taking more than you need or more than is freely offered

Asteya is about not stealing or taking anything that doesn't belong to us, but its focus goes beyond material possessions. Asteya looks at all levels of our being. The capitalist perpetuates the idea that more is better, that bigger is better and that there is greater value attached to possessing more capital. Asteya challenges us to be mindful in our choices around what we consume, take, need and desire.

Aparigraha: non-possessiveness, non-grasping, letting go of attachment

Aparigraha builds on the intent of Asteya. It encourages one to assess unhealthy attachments, negative thinking or old belief patterns, fears, and desires. Dominant culture thrives because of a belief in scarcity. Aparigraha invites one to believe in abundance.

Brahmacharya: energy management, managing extremes, cravings, specifically sexual energy

Brahmacharya is composed of two parts. The first is the root "car", which means, "to move." The second is brahma, which means, "truth." Brahmacharya is the movement towards essential truth.

Niyamas (Restraints):Ethical behavior towards ourselves

Saucha: purification, cleanliness in body, mind, and emotions

Saucha means "cleanliness." The yoga asanas and pranayama are an essential means through which we can attend to inner and outer saucha.

Santosha: Contentment

Santosha is the practice of acceptance. When one is clear about the truth of the moment they can ask themselves what is within their power to make necessary changes for the greater good.

Tapas: will, passion, perseverance, heat in the practice

Tapas is one of the most powerful concepts in the Yoga Sutra. The word "tapas" comes from the Sanskrit verb "tap" which means, "to burn." The traditional interpretation of tapas is "fiery discipline." In order to create a just world, one needs perseverance, passion to create new ways of being.

Svadhyaya: self-study, absorbing spiritual wisdom, non-judgmental self-observation

Svadhyaya is the practice of self-reflection. This practice allows one to see themselves more clearly and to connect with the divine within, which will allow them to see the divine spark that exists in all beings.

Ishvara Pranidhana: surrender to God or Spirit, offering the fruits of your actions up to something greater.

Ishvara Pranidhana means to surrender to a higher source to "lay all of your actions at the feet of God/the Divine." In moving closer to the Divine, one is able to work towards a higher purpose focused on the oneness of all beings.

The yamas and niyamas offer a framework for how to create a just world.

The Role of Feelings

Emotions override thoughts. Every time. The practice of yoga beckons us to notice our feelings. It invites one into a practice of quieting the mind enough to feel the most subtle emotions and sensations. Yoga allows us to connect with the energy body - our spirit - and to move from the most dense outlayer -our skin - to the deepest inner layer our soul, or atma. Dominant culture values intellect over emotion, rational thought over feelings. Our culture conditions us to notice what is going on from the head up and not from the throat and heart down. The only way out is through, by way of the feelings. If we are going to make social change, we need to cultivate a practice of feeling. If someone could think us out of the social injustice that we are swimming in, a very smart someone would have done so by now. When one connects with their feelings as yoga teaches us to do, they can connect with their heart. If one is connected with their heart, they have the opportunity to be changed and to shift their perspective. They have the opportunity to feel the pain of living in a world that is designed to break the spirit through violence, oppression and injustice. Feeling the pain, individually and, more importantly, collectively allows for us to grieve, to acknowledge and truth tell and to aspire to be better than the legacy that white supremacy has left us.

Love

"The practice of love offers no place of safety. We risk loss, hurt, pain. We risk being acted upon by forces outside our control."

— bell hooks, All About Love: New Visions

As I began my own journey into actively training folks about racism, my co-trainer and mentor, Tema Okun, told me that anti-racist work requires love. She told me that I would have to love white people to do this work and that I would have to love myself in a world that has taught me to do the opposite. I was confused when she offered this advice about love. I considered myself an awake, conscious, compassionate and loving person. What she was saying was something much deeper. She was suggesting that it is impossible to separate love from anti-racism work. Love needs to be at the center of the work. It is an act of loving care to engage in social justice work.

I also believe it is an act of love and care to move people in their bodies. When we teach, we are inviting people into a loving conversation with themselves and their internal environment so that they might express that love outwardly to the beings they encounter. It is difficult to love in the face of hate. It is difficult to love when one is being made invisible by another. It is difficult to love when one's truth is being questioned and doubted. Love is about seeing your own humanity and the humanity of others. It is about collective care. To lead a practice of social justice through yoga one must make a commitment to revisit and recommit to love again and again. If we practice and center love we have a chance at changing things. We can create a just world. If we distract from love then we are just that -- distracted -- while white supremacy, oppression and hate thrive. May we love our way into being the just world that we can be.

Our Call to Action

We are living in a space where our lives depend upon our shared humanity in a way that I haven't ever experienced in my 41 years on this planet. White supremacy and capitalism are coming for all of us. If we don't begin to consider how our thoughts, words and actions impact the collective good, we will perish. If we don't begin to work collectively and in solidarity with one another, we will perish. The journey of discovering that our dharma is connected to the greater good is challenging and we must do it anyway. We must skillfully take collective and radical action to create a world that allows all of us to breathe, be, live, be seen and validated.

Skill in Action Practice #1

As you embark on this journey with me it is important for you to consider where you come from as a person, and as a racialized being.

Where are you From is based on George Ella Lyon's poem "Where I'm From." It has been used as a template in many settings and I offer it here as a structure for you to consider how you would define where you come from and how you came to be.

You may use the template or not. It is here as a guide for you.

George Ella Lyon

Where I'm From

I am from clothespins, from Clorox and carbon-tetrachloride.

I am from the dirt under the back porch. (Black, glistening,

it tasted like beets.)

I am from the forsythia bush the Dutch elm whose long-gone limbs I remember

as if they were my own.

I'm from fudge and eyeglasses, from Imogene and Alafair.

I'm from the know-it-alls and the pass-it-ons, from Perk up! and Pipe down!

I'm from He restoreth my soul with a cotton ball lamb and ten verses I can say myself.

I'm from Artemus and Billie's Branch, fried corn and strong coffee.

From the finger my grandfather lost to the auger, the eye my father shut to keep his sight.

Under my bed was a dress box spilling old pictures, a sift of lost faces to drift beneath my dreams.

I am from those moments--snapped before I budded --leaf-fall from the family tree.

Template

Where I Am From Poem

Use this template to draft your poem, and then write a final draft to share on blank paper.

I am from _____ (specific ordinary item)

From _____ and _____ (product name) (product name)

I am from the _____ _____ (home description) _____ , _____ , _____ __ (adjective) (adjective) (sensory detail)

I am from _____ _____ , (plant, flower, natural item) _____

_____

_____ (description of above item)

I'm from _____ and

_____ (family tradition)

(family trait)

From _____ and

_____ (name of fam-

ily member) (another family name) I'm from

the _____ and

_____ (description of family tendency)

(another one)

From _____ and

_____ (something you were told as a

child) (another) I'm from _____ ,

_____ (representation of

religion or lack of), (further description)

I'm from _____

_____ (place of birth and family ancestry) _____

_____ , _____

_____ (a food item that represents your family) (another

one)

From the _____

_____ (specific family story about a

specific person and detail)

Skill in Action Practice #2

You have an understanding of where you are from, now connect your roots with what your heart most desires.

My Heart's Desire

For this practice you will need your journal and the object that you have chosen to use for the Skill in Action process.

We will start with a breathing practice to quiet your mind.

Find a comfortable seat, or, if you prefer you can stand or lay down. Place your object next to you or near you.

To find a comfortable seat, you might want to elevate your hips by sitting on a cushion or pillow or blanket.

Close your eyes or look at the ground in front and begin to breathe into your body. Start by taking deep breaths in and out. Begin to feel the shape change in your body as you breathe in and out. Notice the expansion as you breathe in and the contraction or release with your exhale.

Now, continue to breathe and begin to match the length of your inhale and exhale. This is equal part breathing and can help with clarity and quieting the mind.

Sit for at least three minutes practicing equal part breathing.

Notice the physical sensations and the emotions.

Bring your awareness to the object and notice your connection with it and the energy that it is offering to you now.

Now, bring your awareness to what your heart desires for the world, for healing, wholeness and justice for all beings.

In your mind, using the energy of your object begin to craft a prayer, wish, hope or intention that speaks to your heart's desire. To begin with, just let the words flow.

Once you feel ready to move out of meditation, with each breath cycle bring your awareness back to the expansion and the contraction/release. Return to the space by opening your eyes and picking up your journal.

Write down your prayer for the world, for healing, wholeness and justice for all beings.

For example:

Dear Highest Self,

I want to help create a world where I am fully seen and valued, where I am able to fully see and value all beings and the various identities that they walk with in the world.

I want to work to create spaces that are focused on seeing my own humanity and my higher purpose for the collective good, for all beings. I will create spaces focused on connecting others to their shared humanity by building relationships and community. I will be aware of my identities and how they are affecting a space and my experience and use this awareness to understand that there are multiple truths that exist. I will make space for multiple truths to be expressed and heard. I will make space that is liberatory in nature and focused on freedom and justice for all beings.

Make sure that you include yourself in your prayer, wish, hope or intention. After all, you are going to work to make it a reality.

Now read over your prayer three times.

Take a moment to notice how you feel in your heart.

Chapter 2

What Skill in Action is Not

Now you understand what Skill in Action is and where it comes from. What you must also understand is what it is not.

Intent and Impact: There is a difference

Intentions are great and fine and most people have positive conscious and even unconscious intentions most of the time. But it is important to remember that we do not have control over how our good intentions are experienced by others. In other words, intent does not translate into impact. Meaning well does not translate to not taking personal responsibility.

Mantra: My good intentions are not enough.

Privileged Resistance

Resistance shows up in almost every anti-oppression training that I lead. It shows up in social change work. Many yoga teachers refer to it as part of the process of learning to listen to our bodies as we move through the practice of yoga. It is important to understand when it is showing up and how to respond. It is also important to note who has the option to resist and who doesn't. In anti-racism work, resistance by white people is a manifestation of white supremacy and it actively upholds white supremacy.

It is not skillful to stand in a space of rigidity and resistance. It is not skillful to deny the truth about what we know in our bones. It is a privilege and luxury for some to take space to resist the reality and cultural context, while others suffer at the hands of oppression.

We live in a culture that affirms whiteness, white culture, and racial purity. Most people in the white group have no awareness of their capacity to move in space freely because of how whiteness operates in culture. Whiteness was constructed for social and political reasons. It has changed over time based on the goals of white supremacy-divide and conquer. White skin gives people, white people, a pass. A lack of awareness on white people's part about whiteness as a cultural context, allows for them to be willfully ignorant and to have the privilege of being resistant in a system that teaches them that they are individuals on a level playing field with people of color. Whiteness derails racial justice, because white people can stay in a space of being defensive while people of color are struggling to survive and respond to a system that wants to annihilate us.

Spiritual Bypassing: It's not ok

Spiritual Bypassing comes in many forms. In social justice, spiritual bypassing takes on the idea that "we are one" and uses it to avoid deepening any conversations around the impact of our actions and the responsibility that we have to use our available resources to create a just world.

In yoga, this shows up in individuals and groups who commit to the spiritual practice of yoga but have no awareness of how to live yoga outside of a yoga space, like a studio or a retreat or workshop or teacher training. This makes it very difficult to create authentic relationships that are not focused on our sameness or oneness of being but instead those that allow space for difference. Dominant culture prefers that we focus on our sameness so that it doesn't have to account for the ways that it others people based on difference.

It is important to focus on differences, be able to fully see and experience someone.

I want to believe that we are one, we are connected and we have similarities that speak to our shared humanity. But the reality of my lived experience is that I am different, and that in fact, I am not part of the so-called "one."

There are ways to unify in spite of these differences but they go beyond allowing me and those like me, an entry into a space or a seat at the table. Inclusivity isn't enough. It doesn't equalize or neutralize the experience of holding multiple oppressed identities.

Spiritual bypassing perpetuates the idea that the belief "we are one" is enough to create a reality where we are treated equally and as one. It is not. Spiritual bypassing permits the status quo to stay in place and teaches people that if you believe in something and have good intent that is enough. It is not. Many yoga studios and centers have the intention of creating a space that is accessible to everyone. They may feature murals on their wall with the words like: "We are the oneness of all being." They might go on to have meditation and or dharma classes focused on self-love and compassion. Teacher trainings often focus on training students to understand the 8-limbed path of yoga, which outlines the structure and foundation of the practice. Some studios hold fundraisers and community classes are also common. Yoga studios and centers engage in spiritual bypassing by stopping at setting good intentions while detaching from the important practice of exploring the intersection of social justice and yoga.

Spiritual bypassing allows yoga spaces to suggest that we should live by the tenants of the practice of yoga without considering how to take the teaching a step further. This step includes inviting yogis to think carefully about how so much of what we are experiencing as a collective results from injustice, capitalism, an abuse of power and oppression.

I absolutely believe in the capacity of yoga to make positive and transformative change in the world. But, seeing our goodness internally without feeling a responsibility to the collective whole limits the intention and potential impact of the practice of yoga.

Spiritual bypassing creates an environment that lacks an analysis about how power and privilege relate to the practice of yoga. If the business of yoga doesn't examine its own biases and contributions to injustice, then it denies its own participation in the current cultural climate and reality. Yoga equips practitioners to do more than advance their own practice for personal gain, self-righteousness and personal development. Yoga prepares us to understand what is happening internally so that we can decide how we want to be in this world outwardly, while also recognizing our connection to all beings. If one is truly connected to themselves and the practice of yoga, there is no separation between their internal reality and the external reality.

Yoga encourages a space for deep exploration, curiosity and reflection. The practice asks one to look inside and view their experience as a witness. A practice of witnessing allows one to understand that most places where yoga is practiced are a microcosm of the larger culture. Whatever is happening outside of the yoga space is happening inside of the space. The business of yoga isn't void of power and privilege and the manifestation of how power moves in dominant culture is reflected by a lack of building community when teaching a class, the sequence that is taught, the decor of the studio and the demographic of people practicing. The practice of merging the internal and external reality would allow people to live their yoga. Discernment follows witnessing, which can create a space for one to reflect on their impact on the collective good. Or, their perpetuation of power and privilege to harm the collective good.

We must ask our yoga students and patrons to do more than show up to practice asana on their mat. Yoga teachers, studio owners, and practitioners have a responsibility to notice how injustice in the world is landing in their body and heart. They have a responsibility to talk about alignment in the body and not just from a physical standpoint. True alignment of the body, mind, heart and spirit cultivates wholeness and humanity. When one is misaligned, they are unable to witness or practice discernment. The teachings of the 8 limbed path of yoga focus on principles that can be responsive to the injustices that are happening in the world. They call practitioners into action, by suggesting that the only way to be on the path to enlightenment and the only way to practice yoga is to be compassionate and not cause harm to others. The only way not to cause harm is to understand one's power and privilege and to understand that suffering is perpetuated by a lack of recognizing the imbalance of power in our culture.

Why Yoga has Avoided the Conversation about Power and Privilege

Whiteness

White supremacy is nuanced and insidious. It impacts every part of our culture and its presence is often unstated. Yoga has avoided the conversation about power and privilege because to enter into that conversation means a deep exploration of the intersection of white supremacy and yoga must occur. When white people are asked to look at their own whiteness and supremacy they often become defensive. White people haven't been conditioned to look at themselves as white. They haven't been asked to examine their whiteness or how whiteness is equated with power. Since most of the people practicing, profiting and benefiting from the practice of yoga are white, the norm is to simply avoid a discussion about how that came to be. What is seen as normal is for yoga in the West to be a white exercise class. Yoga avoids the conversation about whiteness, power and privilege because the dominant culture avoids the conversation about racism, oppression, white supremacy and privilege. White people haven't been equipped with the conditioning or skills to name whiteness or to understand how their whiteness is affecting others. It isn't profitable to acknowledge that whiteness exists. The business of yoga doesn't see itself benefiting from an honest conversation about power and privilege and this lets white people off of the hook. And if a white person does begin to examine their power and privilege they have the option of leaving the discussion at any time. People of color aren't afforded that same opportunity.

Capitalism: The Exclusionary Business of Yoga

We live in a capitalist culture that is focused on the sum gain of any action. Yoga hasn't transcended this reality. Put simply, the westernization of yoga appropriates elements from a practice and culture and uses them for financial gain. This often occurs without an awareness of the historical oppression of the groups of people who created yoga. The intersection between capitalism and the business of yoga produces a framework for how yoga looks, defines "yogi" and decides who is more deserving of the practice. The current business of yoga doesn't reflect the cultural reality. Yoga spaces don't reflect spaces that are diverse, welcoming or accessible. They lack diversity in shape, size, race, ethnicity, gender expression and identity, unless it benefits them financially.

The business of yoga perpetuates institutional and cultural oppression. Institutional oppression is based on policies and procedures that exclude, under serve, exploit and oppress people who do not fit the cultural idea of what is normal. People who embody identities that are othered by dominant culture (people of color, persons with disabilities, lesbian, gay, transgender and bisexual people, poor people, immigrants and other marginalized groups) aren't experiencing the behaviors of the institution in exactly the same ways but they are experiencing an invisibilization and invalidation from the institution.

A very clear example of invalidation and invisibilization by the institution is the representation of yoga through the media. For years, I subscribed to Yoga Journal. After graduating from yoga teacher training program I thought that the magazine might help me in learning more about anatomy, yoga poses and the practice of yoga. Cover after cover had a white woman holding a posture that wasn't reflective of the way my body moved or how my body looked. Every once in a while there would be a woman of color or a man on the cover. I didn't see myself in the magazine and the experience of not seeing someone who looked like me in a magazine that currently, reaches tens of thousands of yogis made me understand very clearly who yoga is for: skinny white women. The topics within the magazine rarely focused on social justice issues let alone oppression and privilege.

Yoga Journal is part of constructing the narrative and norms for yoga and those norms are reiterated in many yoga spaces. "The personal is political" is a term that was popularized in the 60s and comes from the feminist movement. The term was originally written about as a response to the notion that "consciousness raising" is actually "therapy." This notion was a response to women gathering to discuss the ways they were being affected by oppression. *The personal is political* means whatever we are experiencing personally is connected with the political landscape. When we are experiencing oppression it is not our individual problem, it is a systemic problem connected to the political context.

When people enter our studios and attend our classes, they are coming with all of the identities they embody, which calls us to respond to them as beings who are navigating a culture that perpetuates systemic oppression.

Yoga and Politics: It's Personal

Yoga has the power to alter how someone experiences themselves. It has the capacity to reveal new insights. Yoga can inspire one to take risks and to grow. It can motivate one to commit to a daily practice, which is a commitment to themselves and their personal transformation. Yoga has saved me time and time again. My mat became the safest space for me. It became a ritual for me to inhabit the four corners of my yoga mat for my own salvation. I have cried and laughed on my mat. I have pushed beyond self-imposed limits and learned to listen to my body. The practice of yoga taught me how to quiet my mind and led me to breathe deeply, connecting me to my true nature and essence. My yoga mat became the safe haven when my black body felt under attack. My yoga mat allowed me to remember to always dedicate my efforts and the energy I expend in the practice to something outside of myself, something bigger than me. Yoga engenders internal transformation. In this sense, it is about the personal, but not void of the connection of the person with the larger culture.

As a teacher, the practice allows me to create space where people are encouraged to be fully themselves. Yoga builds community, changes hearts and invites us to evolve into the best version of ourselves individually and collectively.

After the 2017 election, I noticed that my classes were packed with people wanting inspiration, guidance, and a safe place to be and feel. The collective trauma my students experience and the misalignment of the practice of yoga with the current political landscape called them into a political action through meditation, asana, and dharma discussions. The larger cultural context and how people are experiencing it connects the personal internal transformation with the political terrain.

Yoga is personal and political.

Many studios shy away from becoming involved with political or social justice issues. Remaining neutral in the name of the equanimity is yet another example of spiritual bypassing. Studios feel that they need to remain unbiased in the spirit of accessibility without any analysis or understanding of how yoga as an institution perpetuates bias and oppression. When people avoid social justice and political conversations, they are having a different conversation. A conversation that further marginalizes people who have been historically invisibilized, invalidated and discounted. Studios who focus on being non-biased perpetuate the homogenization of yoga.

The westernized practice of yoga has avoided the conversation about oppression and privilege because it sees itself as a practice that transcends dominant cultures toxic narratives and norms.

It sees itself as an all-inclusive practice doing good for the mind and body without a need to reflect and study the ways in which it is perpetuating cultural and institutional oppression.

Mantra: Skill in action is a practice of recognizing my own and others identities, wholeness and humanity and owning my responsibility to the collective good. Skill in action is truth telling and engaging in the conversation about oppression and yoga. Skill in action is a way of life and being.

Skill in Action Practice #3
Uniquely Positioned

You will need:

- A journal
- Your heart's desire prayer
- The object that you have chosen to use for the Skill in Action process.

During this practice you are going to connect with your internal fire and drive, tapping into your capacity to create change in the world. This is an exploration of recognizing your identities without blame or shame but from a place of truth and self-study.

We will start with a breathing practice to quiet your mind.

Find a comfortable seat, or, if you prefer you can stand or lay down. To find a comfortable seat, you might want to elevate your hips by sitting on a cushion or pillow or blanket. Place your object next to you or near you.

Close your eyes or look at the ground in front of you and begin to breathe into your body. Start by taking deep breaths in and out. Begin to feel the shape change in your body as you breathe. Notice the expansion as you inhale and the contraction or release with your exhale.

Bring your awareness to your chosen object and notice your connection with it and the energy that it is offering to you now.

Now, begin to breathe in and out of your nose, connecting to your ujjayi breath, victorious breath. As you breathe in and out of your nose you will notice that you can hear the sound of your breath and you will feel the sensation of the breath moving on the back of your throat. The ujjayi breath will start to build some heat in the body.

Remind yourself of your heart's desire and your prayer.

Begin to notice all of the identities that you embody: Black, woman, daughter, sister, and yoga teacher, educated...

Take a few more deep breaths and then come back to the space.

Draw a line down the middle of your page and on the left side of the page you will write all of the identities that came to mind during the meditation. On the right side of the page list all of the privileges or ways that you are targeted because of your identities.

For example:

Identities	Privileges or Oppression
Black	• Targeted because of systemic racism by every institution in the U.S.
Woman	• Targeted because of systemic sexism by every institution in the U.S. Invisibilized, not heard, not seen. Underpaid and undervalued
Educated- Masters Degree	• I am afforded the privilege of having access to certain spaces, jobs and conversations because of my level of education
Middle Class	• I can afford to make financial decisions without living paycheck to paycheck. I have access to housing, transportation, food and the many opportunities afforded to someone who has financial means.
Able Bodied	• I am privileged by my mobility. I don't have to think about not having access to a building or space because I can walk and physically move freely.
American	• I am a U.S. citizen which allows me not to be concerned about possible deportation.

Lastly, take a moment to consider how based on your identities you are uniquely positioned to engage with the practice of yoga to create change.

This is what I wrote: I am a black, female yoga teacher. My body being in space as the teacher is revolutionary and is counter to the cultural conditioning about who practices yoga in the West. I am educated, which gives me access to certain spaces. I had the ability to pay for yoga teacher training and from that have been able to teach in studios. Access to teaching has allowed me to take free yoga classes and to be exposed to various teachers. Given that I have access to various yoga spaces, it is my responsibility to actively call people into action by asking them to dedicate each practice to something bigger than them. In addition, I try to access the yoga spaces where I teach to call students into something other than asana practice, I talk about alignment in their bodies and then in the world in their relationships, I discuss the breath being our true nature. I share about narratives that we build and create that limit us and keep us separated from others and ourselves.

Do this practice every day for three days and then on the fourth day, start to write down actions you think you can take within or outside of your community to make change.

CHAPTER 3

BUILDING SKILL IN ACTION

"If you have come here to help me, you are wasting your time. But if you have come because your liberation is bound up with mine, then let us work together."

— Lila Watson

What I know for sure about building Skill in Action and creating a just world

"Two or three things I know for sure, and one of them is that if we are not beautiful to each other, we cannot know beauty in any form."

— Dorothy Allison

D orothy Allison inspired me and a group of anti-racism trainers to develop an exercise entitled, "What I Know for Sure." We used this exercise to bring together a group of anti-racism activists to share lessons learned from their experience working across lines of difference.

I believe that we have to be beautiful to each other in order to experience or know beauty in any form. As a collective, we need to engage in the practice of creating a vision for a beautiful and just world. After leading many yoga classes and countless anti-racism trainings, I know it is important to keep my ego out of my work and to let my heart lead the practice. I know that I am continuing work and standing on the shoulders of many social justice spiritual warriors who came before me. I know that many will come after me and continue this work. The practice of creating justice and teaching yoga will change you in ways that reveal both your shadow and light sides. The worst parts of myself have been exposed as well as the most beautiful and vulnerable parts. The work of creating justice in the world is ongoing and lifelong. In order to make the real change that is needed one must commit to the process and the learning.

The individuals and the collective have to be willing to make mistakes and learn from them along the way. Teaching, discussing or leading a process focused on the intersection of social justice and yoga is messy. Racism is messy. Oppression is messy. Privilege is confusing and messy. Be willing to make a mess. Be willing to sit in the discomfort and the dissonance that so often arises when we are engaged in deep learning. Discomfort is the key to transformation.

Lastly, I know that this work is difficult. No one said that talking about social justice and yoga would be easy. For this reason, many people choose to avoid the conversation. We have to explore these issues. If we do not, we are doing a disservice to all of our yoga students who are yearning to do more with their practice than focus on their own individual needs. As teachers we have the power to call people into a deeper practice.

"Woke"

After the election I noticed that many white people became vocal about the injustices in the world. An awakening of sorts happened. Many people of color have been "woke" and waiting on white people to understand that white supremacy is a cultural condition creating a reality for groups of people that is oppressive and unjust.

Because of the increase in people who were awakened, a yoga studio invited me to facilitate a group discussion for people to share about their feelings in response to the election. The studio is not my home studio; in fact I had never been there. I put away my cell phone, and I missed a call from a dear friend of mine who was dying. Cynthia Brown, a beloved and dismantling racism colleague, was transitioning from this physical plane to another. She had pancreatic cancer.

After she was diagnosed she said to me, "White supremacy is killing me. Cancer and white supremacy are one in the same. They are silent, they grow, it is taboo to discuss them and capitalism intersects with both." It struck me when she said those words to me. White supremacy was killing her and she had to face the capitalist system to receive treatment for what white supremacy had done to her.

The yoga studio was full of white women and a few people of color. We opened the space, chanted Aum, moved through the evening and ended with another chant focused on all beings happiness and freedom. The space was well intentioned and the call to action was timely but I sat there wondering why it took so long for the yoga community to have a discussion about what led up to the result of the election of Donald Trump as our President.

A white woman shared how she was feeling fired up and ready for action. She expressed feeling like her family would be impacted by the result of the election. She was now personally affected by oppression. She didn't acknowledge the fact that oppression has been present since the inception of this country. Nor the fact that she has been privileged because of other people's oppression.

After she finished speaking I said to her, "I will forgive you for taking so long. I will forgive white folks for taking so long to respond. I've been waiting on you for a very long time."

White supremacy is so adaptable and so powerful that it allowed this woman to be complacent until she felt personally affected. White supremacy allowed for the yoga studio to wait to have a conversation about oppression. White supremacy conditioned that yoga community to escape the effects of oppression. The personal didn't become the political, until she felt personally affected by oppression. Until this moment, she felt unaffected and didn't feel called to respond to the physical and psychic deaths of groups of people who have been historically oppressed since the beginning of time. Yoga taught me to forgive the white woman who sat in that yoga studio inspiring other mostly white women with her words. Yoga taught me to be honest with her about her complacency and my desire to have had her in this conversation long ago. I cannot be let off of the hook; I don't have that privilege. My friend was dying and white supremacy was winning. Spiritual bypassing, cultural appropriation, depending on "being good" as being enough, making personal changes and showing up for the physical practice of yoga causes the yoga community to respond in their own time or not at all.

The yoga community has had the luxury of not participating in conversations about oppression and privilege.

Practicing Skill in Action requires an understanding that we, as a collective group of beings, are inextricably bound by our liberation and our suffering. Dominant culture doesn't support this belief. It assumes that we are individuals living in the world and we don't need to respect or notice the other beings that are living amongst us. It is important to understand that to radical-ize your practice of yoga, you must see the ways in which you aren't liberated and the ways that you are experiencing suffering. Know that whatever you notice about your own experience of liberation and suffering is related to the other ways that all be-ings suffer and experience freedom. As an institution yoga can respond to the reality of our bind to one another by creating accessible spaces and exploring the intersection of the practice of being a justice worker and yoga practitioner.

Creating Accessible Spaces for the Practice of Yoga

As you reflect on your own experience of discovering and prac-ticing yoga, take a moment to examine all of the identities that you embody and how those identities impacted your ability to access the practice of yoga. Think about your socio-economic status and ethnic background and ask yourself:

What has been hard for you because of these things?

How have these things been a source of strength?

How has your background, strengths and challenges intersected with your ability to access yoga?

I felt as if I had everything I needed growing up, but I witnessed my mother struggling to pay bills and being stressed financially most months. Growing up black made me feel isolated at times and I was very aware of not fitting into dominant culture. I felt very different than the children who attended school with me. I internalized that different was the same as bad or wrong.

As far as strengths go, I learned to value sharing with others even if we only had a little. Taking care of the physical body wasn't something that was practiced through exercise or physical movement in my home. No one in my family practiced yoga. It isn't part of my family's cultural background and yoga was cost prohibitive. For my mother, there were many other financial obligations.

When I began to practice yoga in college, the cost was included in my semester's tuition. I just had to show up for the class. All of the props were available in the college gym, so I didn't have to think about buying a mat or purchasing blocks, straps or other equipment. When I joined a gym in graduate school and began to practice yoga, all of the props were in the gym and the classes were included in my monthly membership fee. After becoming a certified yoga teacher, I was able to access yoga spaces without paying for classes because of being a teacher in the studio. If I travel and take classes, often studios offer a discount for yoga teachers. In college, my socio-economic background and ability to take out student loans to attend college allowed me to be introduced to yoga and then to be able to afford to pay for the practice until I became a teacher.

My current socio-economic background has afforded me the opportunity to discover the deep spiritual teachings and experience of yoga. It's important to also reflect on how we are seen and experienced as we enter a yoga space. My privilege as yoga teacher allows me access in some spaces but my identity as a black woman contradicts cultural norms about what it means to be a yogi in this country.

Take a moment to think back to the first time that you entered a yoga class or studio. How did you feel? What did you notice about the space? What stood out about the teacher? Did you feel welcome? How did you feel when you left the class?

How we set up a space and who is allowed to use the space determines everything.

Yoga has great power to shape the cultural norm of what it means to practice yoga as well as the embodiment of being a "yogi." Cultural norms in the yoga studio are reflective of culture as a whole. Dominant, white supremacist culture reflects a general norm of being white, thin, able bodied, and gender conforming.

Therefore, much of what we see in yoga practice spaces reflects these larger cultural norms.

Yoga is touted as a practice that can benefit everyone. Researchers are conducting studies on how effective yoga is in reducing stress and promoting mindfulness. The military has started yoga programs for veterans to address their Post-Traumatic

Stress Disorder. Survivors of sexual violence are being taught yoga to safely move back into their bodies. Yoga is marketed to mothers-to-be, to men who aren't flexible and to pro-athletes. Yoga as a practice is marketed as being accessible when in reality most people who are practicing yoga are white, thin, women, English speaking, heterosexual and middle-to-upper class. Yoga has departed from its roots, intended purpose and has become an exclusive practice.

Yoga allows us to access our innermost emotions, sensations and desires. Yoga helps us access the various layers of self: the ego, spirit and the heart. A yoga space must be conducive to safe reflection and discovery.

Our environment affects us on an emotional level. So often, our environment is reflective of our internal state. Generally speaking, many yoga spaces are set up to create a calm environment that will assist people in quieting their minds. This can translate into spaces feeling like an escape from the outer world, which further focus on individualized self-care and relaxation. Taking care of oneself and learning to quiet the mind are important practices but not as powerful if only practiced in elite spaces.

In my experience, Most studios believe that they are addressing accessibility through their class offerings, physical environment and mission as a studio. To be truly accessible, studios must go beyond beautifying their physical space and offering diverse classes.

It is a very common experience for me as teacher and student, to be the only person of color in the room. I have struggled with what it means for me to be teaching in spaces that are mostly white. I have that same question about what it means to practice in spaces that are mostly white. I believe in my teachings and offerings and it is very difficult to manage teaching from a place of social justice as a black woman in a white space. No one deemed yoga as only for white people and people don't generally talk about white spaces. That is one of the insidious parts of whiteness, it's seen as the norm therefore it is invisibilized as an identity or reality. Because whiteness is often unnamed, it's power to permeate a structure, institution and culture is immense. Since whiteness is seen as the norm in yoga spaces, it leaves little room for creating spaces that are anything other than white, able bodied, female-identified spaces.

To live into the value of accessibility, yoga as an institution must consider:

- Who is being excluded from the practice and the space?

- Who is being included in the space and practice?

- What might prohibit people of various backgrounds from feeling as if this space was for them or a safe place to practice?

- Who is being served through the studio or practice spaces mission or vision for yoga?

- Who is being underserved?

- Who is being oppressed and exploited because of cultural appropriation?

- Is the practice space responsible to the roots of yoga and is it honoring the culture that this practice came from?

- When someone enters this space will they feel a resonance, will they see themselves reflected in the physical environment, teachers and class offerings?

- Is the cost of classes prohibiting groups of people from being able to practice in this space?

These are not easy questions and the answers might be even more difficult to accept, let alone address in some way. These questions are here for one to access the space they are creating and to begin to think about how to create a socially just and aware practice space. While it is difficult to address all of the areas where yoga is lacking in its attempt to be accessible, it is important for one to make changes where they can and to continually sit with these questions, revising their space, offerings and ethos.

Space to Fully be Ourselves

Building a space that allows us to be our full selves requires that the space be committed to allowing people to enter into the space with all of their identities affirmed, seen and supported. Being forced to leave parts of ourselves outside of a space causes fragmentation to the body, mind, heart and spirit.

We live in a culture that promotes fragmentation through cultural values. This culture teaches us to be competitive, over effort, strive, and to push past edges. Dominant culture teaches us to act from the neck up, valuing intellect over emotionality and rational thought over inner wisdom. Living in this culture conditions us to disconnect from our humanity and inner knowing and sometimes to act in a way that isn't in our best interest or in the interest of the collective good.

Based on our interaction with culture, we internalize messages about what it means to embody various identities. I have internalized messages from the toxicity of white supremacy. The same goes for white people. We have taken in different messages and we express our internalizations in very different ways. People of color and marginalized groups internalize messages of inferiority. People who are privileged by the oppression of others internalize messages of superiority. The messages of inferiority and superiority are reinforced by cultural norms.

As a black woman I have internalized that I am stupid, surprisingly "articulate", irresponsible, and that I have to work twice as hard. I have internalized that I am untrustworthy, invisible, worthless and invalid. I received these messages from the institutions with which I interact, and the cultural norms perpetuated by these institutions. I continually get these messages despite receiving very positive messages from my mother and family while growing up.

If I am receiving these messages from culture, the converse is happening for folks who are being privileged by my oppression. They are receiving messages that they are safe, deserving, trustworthy, visible, valid, worthy, smart, better than, and capable. Not everyone benefiting from white supremacy or patriarchy is receiving these messages in the same way, but they are disproportionately internalizing that they are just a little bit better than, people of color, women, LGBTQ people, poor people and other groups who are marginalized by the system.

It is important to build a container and space that allows people to be their full selves so that they can feel and see their humanity. This container allows people to feel fully alive and aligned and to live into values based on creating a just world. The container and space invites people into understanding how their suffering and liberation is bound to all beings suffering and liberation. From a place of alignment, affirmation, wholeness and a belief that a just world can exist, as a collective we can transform the cultural norms that are killing our planet and us.

How to be Inclusive

Yoga is deeper than the postures, clothing worn to practice, music that is playing in the background and the blissful euphoria that people feel every once in a while after a practice. It is possible to practice yoga all of the time, on our mat, in our interactions and through the choices we make in our lives. Let's explore the practical set up of a space for the physical asana practice and then broaden this idea to the larger collective.

Inclusive Branding

Whatever is going on internally is reflected externally. The branding of yoga affects how yoga spaces are set up, how they market their business and who practices in the space. Inclusive branding should include a diversity of people represented in any promotion of the practice of yoga.

This is not an invitation to tokenize any individual. Rather, it is an invitation to let people know that yoga is truly for everyone.

It is important for a yoga space to understand their connection to community. Not just the people in the surrounding neighborhoods but the people whom they would like to benefit from the practice of yoga. A yoga space could create a mission that is focused on inclusion and then review their practices and policies related to marketing and branding to assess how they are or aren't living into their mission.

Inclusive of POC

As a woman of color, it is important for me to feel like the practice of yoga is intended for me and that I can be included in the practice. All of me. I have had the disjointing experience of entering spaces to practice yoga and have immediately lost my breath because of an often unspoken vibe that tell me I am not normal and that I am not what is expected in the space. I have had teachers and studio owners assume that I haven't practiced yoga before. They didn't ask me. They actually told me where to set up so that I can be behind someone so that I can keep up with the sequence. I have been the only person of color in classes and that has made me wonder is this a welcoming place for people of color.

Inclusive Embodiment

Yoga spaces can embody the practice of yoga by being welcoming to everyone, by asking if someone has practiced yoga before and by giving people the agency to set up their mats wherever they want.

Often, I look at the class schedule to see what offerings the studio has and if there are any teachers of color. I am looking for a reflection of myself. If a studio doesn't have teachers of color, I look to see if they have a diversity of classes or workshops that speak to social justice or how we are experienced based on our various identities.

I am curious about whether or not a studio is connected with the community and if their connection to the community is part of their identity as a studio. I look to see if there is a sliding scale or work-study option. Through my lens as a woman of color, I am assessing how authentic and true to the practice a yoga space might be before I ever walk through the door of the space for the first time.

Applying a lens of inclusion to the larger cultural context reminds us that yoga doesn't end when we roll out our mat or when we roll it up at the end of the physical practice. Yoga is truly a lifelong practice that has the power to influence who we are in the world. Think about who you are in the world. Who do you interact with on a regular basis? If you are in a work setting, who is included in your organization? Whose voices are valid and valuable? Whose narrative is being uplifted and who is being resourced? Who is profiting off of the work that you do in the world and is the way you do your work related to the values of the practice of yoga, justice, fairness and inclusion? If one wants to live into the practice of yoga on their mat and in their lives they must be aware of the privilege they walk with and how their privilege means that another group of people is being oppressed, excluded and made invisible.

Building a Safe Space for Yoga

As a yoga teacher and social justice activist, I do many things to make sure that I can build a safe container for students. I have my own practice of yoga, meditation and centering, which allows me to show up more fully for others. Moving through my own centering practice prepares me to be fully and deeply present with others. When I am present, I am able to "tune into" energy, the presence of others through their body language and words. Once I tune into what is going on in the space, I can fully listen and notice what is occurring on the surface and under the surface. The skill of centering preparing, being present and listening creates an environment that feels safe to others. People feel held and seen in the space and they are able to show up, as they truly are, the messiness and the beauty. A space where others can show up as they truly are requires me to be authentic and vulnerable. I am mindful of what I share with students and only share if I believe it will be in service of their growth. Mindfulness around what to share and how defines how much space I take up. The practice of yoga and social justice are sacred to me on their own and as they intersect with one another. I create a safe and sacred space. Creating a safe space is about compassionate authentic connection. I strive to create this environment in every interaction and setting. Trust is built from there.

As one considers how to create a safe space or build a safe container reflect on how you do the following:

- Practice what you offer
- Consent
- Use Language
- Offer cues and modifications
- Adjustments
- Silence

Practice

One of my colleagues who leads Dismantling Racism Trainings with me always says that she is an anti-racist and she is a racist. I appreciate that she understands that she hasn't learned all that there is to learn about anti-racism work. She understands that she needs to continue to practice. She knows that there is a shadow side and a side that is striving to make this world a better place. I am a better teacher in all things when I am practicing what I am offering to others. When I am not practicing understanding how I am internalizing negative messages from culture about my race, and how those messages are affecting me, I cannot be in a place of compassion and practice self-care. When I don't practice yoga, meditation or a centering practice, I am not the best teacher that I can be. I can feel it in my body and soul. If I haven't practiced, I feel uninspired by what I am offering and teaching. Develop a practice for yourself. This can include a meditation, ritual, breathing activity, asana practice or a walk outside to be in the expanse of nature. Practice so that you can show up fully for your students and yourself.

Building Trust

Consent

At its best, the practice of yoga makes a person feel like they have complete agency over their bodies and the choices they make around how to move. When people are given fewer choices and discouraged from paying attention to their own intuition about their bodies and emotional state, they aren't able to cultivate confidence in their ability to know what is best for them. Dominant culture requires us to interact with institutions and organizations that decide things for us based on our identities.

So often we aren't able to shape our own narrative about assumptions and ourselves lead people to actions that may not be in our best interest.

In the yoga space, there are many ways that we can offer consent to students through our use of language, cueing, modifications and adjustments. When students leave my classes or trainings, I want them to feel like they created their experience of the practice. I want them to feel as if they were welcomed and supported by my words and actions.

Use of Language-gender assumptions

Language is powerful. It shapes narratives and norms. Language can create connection or isolation.

I have been in countless classes where the teacher says, "We are all women here," or "Ladies, you know what it's like when..." A few years ago I attended a pre-natal, post-natal workshop and the assumption there was that all couples are heterosexual through language that suggested that mothers are stressed out and trying to recover from birth and fathers cannot possibly know all that a mother is going through.

Yoga through a social justice lens requires yoga studios to understand that people who are gender non-conforming or identify as lesbian, gay, transgender or bisexual don't need us defining their gender identity, sexual orientation or gender expression for them. As an institution, yoga must move away from language that categorizes people and takes away their agency to be their full self. Avoid generalizing to create a space that is inclusive and affirming. Speak for yourself using "I" statements and assume that you don't know anything about how people identify in the class but take the opportunity to welcome everyone. I avoid making any assumptions about gender by leaving gender pronouns out of my cueing.

Foster an environment that is open to all by leaving out the words: beginner, intermediate or advanced. I work around this language by offering options and modifications. If I do offer a more "advanced" variation of a pose, I say, "Notice the breath in your body, let it be your guide and if you want to add to this posture here are your options."

Cueing and Modifications

Cueing, sequencing and modifications are very important. As a teacher or guide, let people know that you will offer modifications or options and encourage individuals to listen to their bodies and hearts more than they are listening to your cues. This gives people the opportunity to practice discernment and to clarify what will best serve their bodies and hearts in the moment. This service to the body and heart isn't just about the individual, it is tied to coming back home to the self to then be able to expand out in service of the larger collective. When people choose to modify or adjust I reinforce that what they are doing is tuning into to their needs and then responding by honoring what they hear as they tune in. In this way, people are taking care of themselves not from a self-centered space but from a space of deep listening.

Adjustments

In my experience, yoga teachers have different ways of addressing adjustments. Some teachers let students know at the beginning of class that they will offer adjustments and to let the teacher know if they don't want one. Other teachers adjust without asking and as a teacher I have had students say no to adjustments. Marginalized groups of people are asked to adjust who they are most of the time. In response to cultural norms people will shift and change in ways that are harmful, unhealthy and not in their best interest. Sometimes people must do this for their own safety and protection.

During the summer of 2017, I was stopped by a police officer two weeks after the police had murdered two black men. The officer followed me for over a mile and then pulled me over. I was wracking my brain trying to figure out what on earth he could stop me for. He walked up to my car and he said that my registration wasn't current. I knew that my registration was in my glove compartment. I started to reach for it and then I froze. I adjusted. I knew that if I moved too quickly that could trigger something for the officer. The cultural backdrop was one where black men were getting murdered while their hands were up or when they informed officers that they had a gun and license for the gun. I am unsure of what the officer would have done had I reached for the glove compartment but I knew better than to move. I sat and explained to him that I thought it was in my glove compartment. I asked permission to reach into the compartment for it and he granted me permission. In the end, he ended up putting my sticker on my license plate for me. This adjustment isn't unfamiliar to me. I adjust how I move, if I move, what I say and how I act to survive in this culture. I don't want to have to be forced to move in a particular way or to be moved or manipulated in yoga class.

To make a safe yoga space, teachers must allow their students to decide whether or not they want an adjustment. This is a place where a teacher can actively practice asking for consent. This can be a verbal exchange or some yoga studios have chips or notes that students can place at the top of their mat to indicate whether or not they want adjustments.

Assuming that adjustments always feel good is dangerous. Yoga has seen the abuse of power via sexism, heterosexism, racism and ableism. There is a history of manipulating and exploiting bodies, and these historical memories are held in our nervous systems in ways that we cannot always understand. Yoga teachers, holding space for students need to be aware of the power of touch and its ability to heal or harm. For your teaching consider how you will ask about adjustments, be consistent about it and always let the class know that the adjustments are optional. Empower the students to make the choice about what they need.

Assess how you are building a safe container and shift what you need to be able to create a space that will allow you and your students to see themselves, thrive and grow into their highest self.

The Use of Silence

The practice of Skill in Action includes the practice of silence. Yoga asks us to go inside and see ourselves, exploring from the inside out. A central part of yoga is sitting in silence, listening to the sound of your breath. Yoga encourages us to move into silence to practice self-reflection, notice patterns and our responses to them and to practice discernment. Dominant culture conditions most of us to fill the space. Reactivity is the norm. This can look like not pausing before you respond or making a decision that lacks inclusivity or transparency. These responses and decisions have consequences for others. Silence creates a space for deep listening, which is central to yoga and making social change. Deeply listening allows for introspection, connection and for relationships to be built. When we are listened to, we are seen and heard. Being seen and heard can make one feel valued and appreciated; like they have a voice that matters. Creating spaces where people's voices matter and influence change for the collective good is an essential part of creating a just world.

Skill in Action Practice #4

Justice in the Body, Justice in the World

You will need:

- A journal
- Your heart's desire prayer
- The object that you have chosen to use for the Skill in Action process.

During this practice you are going to connect your capacity to Build Skill in Action by considering what justice looks and feels like in your body and the world.

We will start with a breathing practice to quiet your mind.

Find a comfortable seat, or, if you prefer you can stand or lay down. To find a comfortable seat you might want to elevate your hips by sitting on a cushion or pillow or blanket. Place your object next to you or near you.

Close your eyes or look at the ground in front of you and begin to breathe into your body. Start by taking deep breaths in and out. Begin to feel the shape change in your body as you breathe. Notice the expansion as you inhale and the contraction or release with your exhale.

Bring your awareness to your chosen object and notice your connection with it and the energy that it is offering to you now.

Now begin to breathe in and out of your nose, connecting to your ujjayi breath, victorious breath. As you breathe in and out of your nose you will notice that you can hear the sound of your breath and you will feel the sensation of the breath moving on the back of your throat. The ujjayi breath will start to build some heat in the body.

Open your eyes and read your heart's desire prayer aloud.

From your heart's desire prayer and your object that represents justice.

In your journal, from your heart's desire prayer write down what justice looks like in your body. What conditions need to be present for you to feel like you are being treated fairly and in a just way? What does it mean to be in full alignment with your values and how do you live out that alignment in the world?

Take a few deep breaths and reflect on what you've written.

Now, go back to your journal and write down a commitment statement focused on creating justice for others in the world. Connect what you've written about alignment and justice in your body with actions you will take in the world.

Take a few deep breaths and reflect on what you've written.

Condense your commitment statement into one sentence. Write this sentence in your journal and on an index card of post it note. Place the index card or post it note somewhere you will see it daily. It will serve as a visual affirmation or cue for you to remember your commitment to yourself and others.

Read your commitment three times a day.

Justice in my Body

Justice in my body feels like the capacity to breathe and move freely in my body and space. Justice in my body looks like me having full control over when and how I give consent. It feels like me being unapologetic for being me and having space to fully express myself. Justice in my body feels like complete alignment physically, emotionally mentally and spiritually.

This relates to the spaces that I create for others cultivating a space for all beings to breathe and move freely.

Statement of Commitment

I commit to creating spaces that allow beings to fully express who they are and to breathe fully and deeply into their very being.

The Nature of Change

Several years ago, I participated in an activity called the "Wave," developed by Stephen Cope and Kripalu. In it, one is asked to hold a yoga posture for five minutes and given some cues for support which include: breathe, relax, notice/feel, allow and watch. It highlights that our bodies can hold most positions for five minutes or more, but our minds get in the way and interrupt us riding the wave of experience. What strikes me about the wave of experience and the accompanying sensations is that the nature of change is like a wave, there is a beginning, middle and end. And then, the next wave. We know this from the asana practice of yoga. If we allow ourselves to stay in a pose for a few more breaths, there is a physical and sometimes energetic release.

The work of creating a just world isn't easy and it takes time. There will be many times when you want to jump off of the wave of experience. If we are able to breathe into our experience acknowledging the injustice in the world, relax where we can and begin to notice our feelings as well as allowing the sensations to be so and then watching so that we can adjust, we have a shot at making lasting change. Arjuna was invited to engage in the war in the same way - to understand his dharma, to breathe and surrender to it, to notice feelings and allow and to witness through the practice of meditation and mindfulness. We can and must make sustainable change.

Holding Space

"Holding space for another person is incredibly profound. When you hold space for someone, you bring your entire presence to them. You walk along with them without judgment, sharing their journey to an unknown destination. Yet you're completely willing to end up wherever they need to go. You give your heart, let go of control, and offer unconditional support.

And when you do, both of you heal, grow, and transform."- Lynn Hauka

The manner in which we set the tone for a space defines the experience that people have within the space. As Lynn suggests, holding space can create an environment ripe for healing and transformation. Conversely, if space isn't held well or irresponsibly it can feel overwhelming and unsafe.

Every time I teach, whether in a yoga class, anti-racism workshop or within the context of working with a private client, I think about my role and how I want the space to be experienced. I have to be mindful of the power I have as a teacher. I am controlling the space. I am setting the tone, creating and delivering the curriculum or sequence and creating a norm in the classroom.

I understand that people are coming from various spaces before they arrive in my yoga class. They may have been caught in traffic, had an argument with a partner, had a rough day at work, just received great news about a new job opportunity or just received relieving news about a health condition that was cause for concern. People come from various spaces and they also enter into the space with a myriad of identities.

Interactions with Students Before and After Class

Caring for a class includes our interactions with students before and after class. The yoga space is for the students and the teacher is responsible for both holding the space and facilitating a process/class that is responsive to the needs of the class. As students enter into a class, teachers can begin holding the space by checking in with new students, acknowledging the returning students and then taking their seat at the front of the class. Allowing space for the students to truly arrive and ground is an important part of the practice of yoga given that people come from very different spaces to land on their mat. Their practice of yoga and the safe space on their mat might be the only moment of solace and self-reflection they receive all day. Since teaching a class and holding a space is an energy exchange between teachers and students, it is important for the teacher of the class to be mindful of the energy that they are taking in before class. If a teacher comes into class after just having a conflict with a friend, it is important to clear that energy, otherwise it could end up showing up in class and that isn't fair to the students.

At the end of class after moving people out of savasana and back into a comfortable seat, I instruct the class to consider what they received from the space, the breath, each other and the practice of yoga. Then, I remind them of the light inside of all them as a reflection of the light inside of me. I let them know that if they have questions they can ask me and I start to pack up my things.

I am available after my class for a few minutes but in general, I am out of the space pretty quickly. I don't ask students for feedback. I trust that if they want to give me feedback, they will do so by never returning to my class or showing up every time I teach. I check in with people who seem like they might need it by asking if they are okay. I ask in a way that allows a person to talk to me if they choose to but that doesn't require them to tell me anything. I would never want to put pressure on a student or open up something for them that I cannot responsibly close in the context of the yoga space. The model of showing up, letting the students arrive and settle, leading them through an experience and then closing the space lets the students know that I am there for them, to teach, to hold space and to remind them to breathe. I am not their guru, their therapist, their friend, their doctor or physical therapist. I am myself in that space, leading a process. Facilitating a process in this way allows students to fill the space in the way that they need, physically and emotionally. There is a routine or ritual around it.

Dharma Talks

Dharma has several translations in sanskrit. It can mean a sermon or speech, a call to action or an expression of someone's duty in the world. In yoga classes, it references a focal point or theme that is shared at the beginning of class by the teacher. These talks are focused on a theme in the world expressed through a personal story from the teacher. In an asana class, dharma talks range between 5-10 minutes. In other contexts, Buddhist teaching or practice dharma talks can last for a much longer amount of time. A teacher may revisit their dharma talk or theme throughout the class. Dharma talks are part of many yoga traditions. Exploring the intersection of social justice and yoga lends itself to making an offering through a dharma talk focused on one's identities and the impact of the oppression and privilege.

When one gives a dharma talk they need to make sure that their sharing is to benefit the class and not themselves or their ego.

If one hasn't checked in with why they are choosing to share they risk ending up processing their own internal issues with the class. If a teacher is in the practice of reminding students of the dharma talk or theme throughout the practice it is important to be mindful of how much space a teacher is filling with their words. For some students, if a teacher shares a lot of personal information about themselves the teacher is seen as more authentic or real. Other students might have the experience of feeling like a teacher is filling up the space with their words and not allowing enough space for self-reflection for the students. More awakening can occur when the teacher isn't filling up the space with their words between each pose or vinyasa.

My willingness to be vulnerable with a class through a dharma talk or other teachings has everything to do with my identity as a woman of color and the fact that mostly white people inhabit the spaces where I teach. In this culture, marginalized groups haven't been encouraged to be vulnerable because in many ways people of color, lesbian, gay bisexual and trans people, people with disabilities, and women's vulnerability has been used against them. For example, when women show emotion they are coded as being overly emotional. When people of color express vulnerability or tender emotion, they are not seen or heard or they are told that they are pulling the race card. Or for me, that I'm an angry black woman. My interaction with students doesn't always involve a dharma talk because in those moments of sharing from a very personal space, I am exposing parts of myself that the culture would rather smother. I offer this background as a way for one to think about how they share information, what they share and what makes it easy or difficult for one to share. Yoga teachers need to be willing to think about the space they inhabit and how they use it and to understand that the ability to move in space is most definitely defined by what one feels entitled to and by one's experience in the world based on their identity.

Self-Care for the Teacher

When I teach and I haven't practiced myself, I feel it and it shows up in my teaching. I feel uninspired, bored with my voice and sometimes I feel resentful because I am offering myself and something to the class that I am in desperate need of myself. It is important for yoga teachers to be practicing, not all in the same way but to have some sort of practice that is grounding, centering and allows for evolution in their teaching. Ask yourself:

If you are a teacher, what do you do to prepare yourself to teach a class or hold space?

What self-care practice do you engage in consistently to help you become a better teacher and practitioner?

It is imperative for yoga teachers to have a practice that marks the end of the class and a self-care practice to release any energy that one might be holding onto from the experience of teaching. I usually walk slowly to my next destination, giving myself time to process and release whatever might still be held in my body and bones from the class. I wash my hands to clear away the physical experience of teaching and to let myself know that I am transitioning. A personalized practice around entering a space and leaving a space is important. If you are a teacher, take time to consider what you will do to care for yourself so that you can continue to teach and keep the energy of the classroom safe and clean. If you are a yoga practitioner, consider how you enter the space and leave it and what energy you might want to take with you once class is over.

Honoring the Roots of the Practice

The Westernization of yoga means that parts of the practice have been rebranded in ways that dishonor the principles of the practice. Businesses profiting from yoga in the West promise weight loss, more money, better sex and more power. Yoga promises to help people find their voice and personal power, to create inner peace and to help practitioners reach a type of enlightenment that makes them void of any accountability or responsibility to other beings. The West has taken yoga. Capitalism has consumed yoga. Yoga has become a business. The consequence is that the history and essence of the practice, the important pearls of the practice are struggling to be retained. Many have simply discarded them.

Cultural Appropriation

Cultural appropriation is the act of taking things from one culture and using them for one's own benefit and material or emotional profit without having any relationship to the people from which they took them. It is hard to live in this Westernized culture without appropriating in one-way or another. To not participate in cultural appropriation, one would have to live in the woods, off the land, naked and without access to material things. Westerners practice of living off of the land began with colonizers taking native land making a holiday called Thanksgiving. They perpetuated white supremacy through the lie that the "Pilgrims and Indians" got along swimmingly and shared an amazing feast. The legacy of theft of land, of cultural norms, traditions and customs lends itself to a culture that appropriates a spiritual practice such as yoga.

Yoga is more than 5,000 years old. It originated in India, but colonization and appropriation have influenced the repurposed practice into what we call yoga in the West. The practice of Hatha Yoga is believed to have begun in the 13th century. In the 17th century, when the British colonized India, practitioners of Hatha Yoga were stereotyped as practicing "black magic," engaging in violent behavior, and perverse sex. Through colonization, the British tried to create more "acceptable" practices of religion. This story sounds familiar.

In the West, the native peoples were seen as savage, inferior to white people and needing to be saved. In the late 18th and early 19th century, the British began working with many Indian administrators and officials to create a modern India, which included a process of "reconciliation" for the native people of India. This included the practice of yoga. Traditional practices were taken and given a Western flare focusing on Western ideals such as the physical body and building a stronger body. A more aerobic version of yoga was born and exported to the West.[1]

Here, we are practicing advanced arm balances, making up postures, focusing on the physical body and building power, getting stronger. While I think all of these things are important, they are void of any spirituality or awareness of anything other than

---

1 Amara Miller, The Origins of Yoga: Part III

one's individual experience. White supremacy culture breeds individualism. It is based on competitiveness, the idea that there is one right way, and receiving benefits based on merit. The exportation, exploitation and colonization of yoga coupled with the ideals expressed in dominant white culture have turned the practice of yoga into an obsession with the purification of the physical body, strength, selfishness and power hoarding all to benefit the individual.

As a teacher, I'm mixed up in this mess. I'm trying to figure out how in the hell I can teach this practice in a way that honors the tradition and pushes people to move past their own individual experience and into a larger consciousness about the collective culture. It is hard to disentangle the practice from colonization in India and what we call the U.S.

It is difficult to disentangle the practice of yoga and the business of yoga in this country and it's nearly impossible to teach in a way that honors the practice. But still, I teach because I believe in the power of the practice. When I show up to teach, I think about my authentic self and how to show up as her. I am aware of the fact that I am practicing something that wasn't mine to begin with but that I benefit from greatly and that I can share with other people. I call people to something bigger through the practice of yoga. I am responsible in my sharing stories about deities, chanting, Sanskrit and sharing principles and beliefs that guide me, but that weren't created by me. I bring in the current cultural context to remind my students and myself that the yoga studio is a microcosm of the outer world. All of the travesties that people experience off of the mat are in the space and every one of us is complicit in the perpetuation of trauma through our actions. We can also choose to be active in our quest towards creating liberation through our actions.

If you are a teacher or studying to become a teacher, take time to notice when you are authentically you.

How do you know that you are showing up as your authentic self?

How do you know when you are taking something from another culture on as your own and sharing it with students without a real connection to the culture?

How does it make you feel? What is within your power to do to show up as your authentic self, to honor the practice of yoga and the culture that it came from?

Skill in Action Practice #5

Multiple Truths

You will need:

- A journal
- Your heart's desire prayer
- The object that you have chosen to use for the Skill in Action process.

Thus far you have focused on your heart's desire for the world, explored your identities and come up with actions that you want to engage in to create a just world. You have meditated on justice in the body and the space that you inhabit as well as thinking about how you can create space for others. Now, I am going to ask you do something that might be a bit more challenging because of how nuanced white supremacy is.

Dominant culture assumes that there is one truth and it generalizes its truth onto everyone. This shows up very directly in the practice of yoga. This generalization also shows up in many other spaces besides the yoga studio or room. I want to teach you a skill that will help you in your interpersonal relationships as well as your relationship with yourself.

You can do this practice anywhere, but it is most effective in a situation that involves someone else and someone who is different than you. They can be different racially, spiritually, emotionally, intellectually etc. This exercise is not about going out and talking to a person that you disagree with or someone whose beliefs will trigger you or traumatize you. So choose your situation very wisely.

During this practice you are going to connect your capacity to Build Skill in Action considering the multiple truths and identities that exist in the world. This will involve you doing some work off of your meditation cushion or mat.

So, choose the situation, a meeting, an encounter at the grocery store, a conversation with a friend. Take a few deep breaths. Remember your commitment to creating a just world.

As you engage with the person that you are sharing space with, I want you to listen to them. I want you to notice what you hear through your own lens based on your identities. I want you to notice the assumptions you make based on how dominant culture defines what is "normal," "right" or "acceptable." I want you to notice emotions and body sensations as you listen to the person you are sharing space with. I want you to consider what you might be missing as a result of viewing things through your lens.

Then, I want you to consider that what the person is really saying, how they are acting and what they are doing is their truth.

Lastly, I want you to practice sitting with your truth and the other person's truth.

Culture teaches us to be either/or, right or wrong and that there is one right way. To create a just world, one must understand that dominant culture white washes things and assumes that all of us are having the same experience at the same time. If you think about it, in reality most people are having very different experiences even if they are in the same setting. The way that one is experiencing something is defined by their identities and lens or framework.

I want you to take your experience of listening for and sitting with multiple truths and journal about what you noticed. And then I want you to practice this skill again. And again. Recording noticings each time. It might be helpful to review your heart's desire prayer and to have your object near you as you journal so that you can feel grounded in your desire to create a just world.

I am usually the one calling out the reality that there are multiple truths and this is a skill I've practiced for years. I first learned about it in Dismantling Racism training when all of us participated in an exercise about our class and ethnicity. In the debrief of the activity the facilitators made the point that they gave the same directions to everyone but all of us had a different experience based on the emotions that we felt at the end of the activity.

Remember that people are having disparate reactions and responses to the cultural conditions. It is skillful to understand this and to hold multiple truths at one time. It is also liberating to sit with multiple truths. It allows for more space.

What you Know for Sure

We will revisit a concept that was introduced earlier in the book: What I Know for Sure. Now that you've been on the path, made your way through this book and contemplated how you too will radicalize the world be clear about what you know; it will ground you as you walk the path.

What I know for sure about yoga and social justice

> *"Two or three things I know for sure, and one of them is that if we are not beautiful to each other, we cannot know beauty in any form."*

> — Dorothy Allison

As you embark on this journey of contemplating how you can radicalize the world through yoga, reflect on what you know for sure about yoga, justice and working across lines of difference.

The prompt:

What I Know for Sure_____

_____.

Make a list of the things you know for sure, post them on your yoga mat, mirror, in your car, in the yoga studio, on social media, anywhere that you will see them. They will serve as a reminder of your dharma.

Vision

"Your vision will become clear only when you look into your heart ... Who looks outside, dreams. Who looks inside, awakens."

— Carl Jung

As you consider what you have learned through the exploration of using your yoga practice to create a just world, you must vision about what kind of world in which you want to live. Change cannot occur without vision, heart, and hard work. So often people say they want to make change in their personal lives or for someone else. If one never envisions the change, then it is very difficult to bring it to life. In my Dismantling Racism work, we end our workshops with people visioning and creating action from that vision. We invite people to move through a visualization where they wake up in a just world. We ask people to notice the sounds, colors, environment, the people, languages being spoken, food being eaten and the life around them. We ask people to pay attention to their role, what part they had in creating the world in which they want to live. I invite you to vision, to dream and to make your dreams and visions come alive. The world in which you want to live is depending on you.

In Africa there is a saying, Ubuntu, which means "I am because you are." Since we are inextricably bound and there is no separation let us be who we are, as a collective, let us be free.

Epilogue

I have memories of standing in my driveway on Whitewood Road in Richmond Virginia, thinking, "Take me away, when are the aliens coming to get me out of here?" I felt out of place and waited for the aliens to save me and take me to some other planetary salvation but it never happened. Now, I understand that I was trying to integrate my identity as a black girl, navigating in a world that saw me as less than, unworthy and invisible. I didn't feel as if the world was made for me and so I wanted to be taken away from it. As a child I was channeling Sun Ra's spirit before I ever learned about him in college during my Introduction to Jazz Class. Sun Ra, named after the Egyptian God of the Sun, believed that he was an alien from Saturn and that his mission on earth was to preach peace. He was a man of color in a country founded on the annihilation of indigenous people and the enslavement and mass murder of black people. He was my predecessor and a fellow lover of the sun. He knew that the consciousness level needed to be elevated for the collective good. Some called him crazy, others called him a revolutionary. I definitely believe he was the latter.

As revolutionaries we must take action.

The world is on fire.

This is a manifestation of the foundation on which this country was built. Colonization, white supremacy, racism and genocide.

At the end of the Gita, Arjuna is asked to release all fear so that he can fully step into his dharma and the path. Krishna believes that Arjuna has successfully moved through obstacles on the pathway to his dharma. He instructs Arjuna to breathe and journey forward.

"Boldness, the ability to lead, large heartedness, courage in battle, energy, stamina, and strength are the natural duties of warriors" -Bhagavad Gita

As I write this, there are protesters in Charlottesville, Virginia rallying against the Unite the Right alt-right white supremacists group. Some of my friends are in Charlottesville in the streets on the front lines, witnessing the vitriolic hatred that comes from a country founded through the means of colonization and genocide. As I browse social media and hear folks around me share their feelings I am struck by how for some the acts of violence occurring right now, as I type, are surprising. Some of my friends are feeling distraught, some are overwhelmed and some are in denial. We cannot afford to continue in this manner. The sole tool of white supremacy is to divide and conquer and that tool is being used effectively and efficiently.

If we do not begin to shift the conversation of yoga to center love, justice and truth-telling then, as a people, we will not survive. As a culture and collective of yogis we must go deeper, dig deeper and use the platform of yoga to create healing, justice and peace.

During this time of political upheaval, cultural genocide through federal policies and practices and a building movement of resistance, we are all Arjuna. We are standing on the battlefield and we are being asked to make a decision about how we will show up as dutiful warriors. We are being called to identify and live into our dharma. The practice of yoga on and beyond the mat can show us how to do just that.

When I work with my students in my teacher training, they leave speaking much more about the anti-oppression training then the actual asana practice they learned to teach. I stress building relationships, creating a shared language and framework and shifting perspectives in my training. This allows participants to dive more deeply and to experience what is underneath the surface of the physical surface and practice. Students have intensified the urgency to respond to injustice, have expanded their definition of yoga and have learned to both regard themselves and others with compassion hearts while also knowing that we must change to make change.

When one learns how to be skillful in action, it is impossible not to take lessons from the yoga room into the world. The overlapping nature of social justice and yoga is apparent when we open our eyes to it. To begin to see requires engaging in self-examination and reflection to understand how our actions, beliefs and words affect others. As a yoga teacher, dismantling racism trainer, social justice activist and human in who is privileged enough to walk in this world, it is my hope that you feel inspired and moved to step up and take action. Justice, liberation and the capacity to breathe in all spaces are our birthright. Let us commit to creating a just world.

May the tears of my ancestors and my own cool the fires and extinguish the flame. May we grieve and rebuild from the ashes and bones of the generations of survivors that came before us. May we as a collective consider what kind of world we will leave for the beings whom will come after us.

May all beings everywhere be happy and free. May our thoughts words and actions contribute to that happiness and freedom for all. May our world be just. May we all find peace.

ABOUT THE AUTHOR

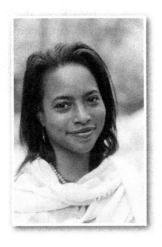

M ichelle is a yoga teacher, social justice activist, licensed clinical social worker and Dismantling Racism trainer. She approaches her life and work from a place of empowerment, embodiment and integration. With a deep understanding of trauma and the impact that it has on the mind, body, spirit and heart, much of Michelle's work focuses on helping people better understand how power and privilege operate in their life. She explores how privilege, power and oppression affects the physical, emotional, mental, spiritual and energy body.

Before yoga, Michelle was a clinical social worker and began her private practice in Chapel Hill, NC in 2001. Michelle specialized in trauma, eating disorders and racial identity work. She has experienced the powerful transformation that comes with embodiment through the practice of yoga. In 2008, Michelle went through yoga teacher training with the goal of infusing different treatment modalities into her practice to better help clients align their minds and bodies. She became a certified yoga teacher in 2009 and went on to complete a 500-hour certification in 2012. In 2015, Michelle began leading her own teacher training: Skill in Action. This training is focused on the intersection of yoga and social justice and it inspires people to consider how they can radicalize their yoga practice to create a just world. Michelle believes in social change and knows that it is her responsibility to embody and inspire change.